Introduction

This reference book to Menopause helps a woman celebrate and honor this natural part of her life. Especially, if she have a good sense of humor.

The reason I chose Australian Bush Flower Essences is because of the wonderful experience I had studying with Dr. Ian White in Melbourne, Australia. Through Dr. White's enthusiasm and knowledge, I have come to know the healing properties of flowers and relish their use.

My classes with Valerie Worwood, and the recipes used from Roberta Wilson's Aromatherapy book, have helped both my client's and myself.

As for Meditation and Healing Affirmations, I have been doing both of these, for years, and have noticed a positive change, within myself, and all that I know who utilize them.

The body is a miraculous healing machine. We just have to allow it to do its work. I hope you enjoy, and most of all, use, the book.

Index

The 25 Most Important Questions About Menopause

More than 50 million baby boomers turned 50 at the close of the 20th century with still one-third to one-half of their adult life ahead of them. Today's woman is hitting her stride, ready to explore universe and expand her activities. You are never too young to learn how to create a first-rate, second half of life for yourself.

Some symptoms of menopause are odd sweats, quirky periods, nervousness, and palpitations. These can be climacteric, between the ages of 45 to 55. This is a new beginning and can be the best time of your life.

WHAT IS MENOPAUSE

Menopause is the end of menstruation and the end of your reproductive years. This process began in puberty with your first period and ends at menopause when your periods stop.

The peri-menopause are those early years of change before menopause where you slow down the production of ovulation and the two female hormones estrogen and progesterone. Post menopause refers to the years after your final period. This is a woman's life rite of passage.

The years between puberty and menopause are a beautifully conducted symphony between the brain and the ovaries. Peri-menopause is the process that begins to add static or to interrupt the music. The *hypothalamus* has the job of producing a hormone that helps conduct the symphony of menstruation. That hormone is *gonadotopin-releasing hormone*. It acts upon the pituitary gland, which in turn, produces other hormones that tell the ovary what to do.

The ovary has two functions: producing eggs and two powerful sex hormones; estrogen and progesterone.

One of the most common symptoms is the hot flash (*vasomotor phenomena*). It is caused when the blood vessels of your skin dilate in an attempt to reset your body's core temperature.

One can avoid hot flashes and night sweats if they avoid alcohol, tobacco, caffeine, spicy foods and stress. Regular exercise and the release of those wonderful endorphin hormones, also help to stabilize your body's temperature. Meditation, guided imagery, biofeedback and visualization techniques can also help. Vitamin E helps many women. One can try 400 IU in the morning and if that does not do the trick, 400 IU in the evening as well.

When estrogen levels decrease, our short-term memory seems to be affected. Urinary tract infections may occur more often.

Other symptoms may include palpitations, insomnia, itchy skin, disorientation, mood swings and even minor depression. Decreased estrogen can make you more vulnerable to stress and stress can exacerbate menopausal symptoms. Lack of testosterone, which women produce in their adrenal glands and ovaries, may cause fatigue.

Follicle stimulating hormone (FSH) is the hormone-determining factor in a woman's blood. The normal amount circulating in your blood during the reproductive years is usually below 40.

There are things that a woman can start as early as her 30's to make her menopause easier. Perform three kinds of exercise that your body requires - stretching for flexibility, weight-bearing exercise to protect your bones and aerobic exercise to protect your heart and lungs.

Quit Smoking. Smoking harms your body and all its functions. Keep caffeine and alcohol to a minimum.

Osteoporosis can occur because bone is living tissue, which continually goes through a natural process of remodeling. Large cells called *osteoclasts* are programmed to discard old bone tissue and replace it with new. After menopause, women who are not on HRT or ERT lose bone at the rate of three percent or more per year.

Natural alternative to hormone are vitamins, minerals and herbs, i.e., potassium and magnesium aspartate, which can improve energy levels. Vitamin E can control hot flashes, vaginal dryness, and some psychological symptoms like mood swings, fatigue, and anxiety when taken with other nutrients like potassium, magnesium, the B vitamins, and bioflavonoids.

You can find Vitamin E in wheat germ, lettuce and green peas and other green vegetables, wheat germ oil and oils made from corn, safflower, sesame, soybeans, and peanuts, grains (brown rice and millet) and mango. Vitamin E is usually not good for anyone with high blood pressure, diabetes, or rheumatic heart condition. High dosages may cause liver problems.

Vitamin B complex is an anti-stress compound. Vitamin B6 in mild doses works as a natural diuretic. Cranberry juice, kelp, watercress and parsley also work as natural diuretics. You can increase your B vitamins by increasing your consumption of beans, and whole grains.

Vitamin C is an anti-stress vitamin. It can also slow excessive menstrual bleeding, speed wound and burn healing and maintain collagen, which is the main supportive protein of the skin, tendons, bones, cartilage and connective tissue. Vegetable sources for Vitamin C are broccoli, Brussels sprouts, cabbage, cauliflower and most greens. Vitamin C can be found in many fruits such as cantaloupe, grapefruit, oranges, strawberries, mango and papaya.

Besides preserving bone, calcium can help us cope with emotional stresses. We need at least 400 IU of Vitamin D to help our bodies absorb calcium. If our calcium intake does not meet those needs, our body will fulfill the need by drawing calcium from the stores in our bones. Every day, we lose between 150 to 200 milligrams of calcium in our urine. The average calcium intake, for the majority of middle aged and elderly women, falls somewhere between 450 and 550 milligrams of calcium per day. When eating rhubarb and spinach, it is necessary to sprinkle them with lemon juice or vinegar to stop the oxalic acid in them from blocking the absorption of calcium into your bones. Another great source of calcium is tofu (the kind made with calcium salts). There is 56 milligrams of calcium in a medium sweet potato and 80 milligrams in three dried figs or one ounce of almonds, and 55 milligrams of calcium in five caramels or six Hershey kisses.

There are a number of herbs that can help with the symptoms of menopause. Chamomile, blackberry root, black cohosh, Dong Quai, passionflower, evening primrose oil and chasteberry are a few. Ginseng is a source of plant estrogen and can enhance energy and relieve hot flashes.

For menopausal insomnia many women take herbal teas, such as, chamomile or catnip. There is also passionflower broth, valerian root, warm milk, warm baths and long evening walks.

Wild Yam has proven useful to women experiencing the symptoms of PMS and menopause. Progesterone taken from the Wild Yam is nearly identical to what our bodies naturally produce.

Guided imagery and relaxation therapy can be used to inhibit hot flashes. They both can help relieve stress and tension as well as combat menopausal symptoms by relaxing from head to toe.

Visualization is another technique where you can create your own atmosphere and environment.

Yoga, when practiced correctly, can enhance muscle and joint flexibility and help to maintain healthy bones.

Biofeedback is a technique that involves being hooked up to a machine that can help to painlessly train our minds to control our heart rate or tension on our muscles.

Acupuncture involves the insertion of hair like fine needles, at certain points on the body's meridians, for the purpose of unblocking our energies.

Massage therapy runs the gamut from reducing stress to bringing relief from muscle strains to relieving stress induced headaches and stiff neck to removing toxins from the body.

Massotherapy is the placement of digital pressure at the same points on the body's meridians (pathways connected to specific organs and body functions) to release the body's energies.

Trigger point therapy pinpoints congestion in the muscles and works with digital pressure to relieve it.

There is relief to be found with iced drinks sipped during the day, cold showers, dressing in layers, eliminating caffeine, alcohol, and spicy foods, and trying to limit stress.

A previously healthy sexual relationship has a good chance of surviving menopause and aging and may even thrive as a result. Studies show that 90% of postmenopausal women surveyed report a complete return of sexual desire. At midlife, take the time to be creative and invent new sexual excitement for yourself and your partner.

At midlife, we should eat better and less then we have before. After the age of 25, our metabolism begins to show down, one half to one percent per year. Menopause, on average at age 51, makes the metabolism more than 25 percent slower than it was. As a woman ages, her percentage of body fat goes up and her percentage of lean body mass tends to go down.

Food is important for our health and our strength; food comes complete with its own pharmacy. The purpose of eating fiber is to have it move through your system and clean it out. Many cereals, especially the bran ones, contain fiber. Most food from plants - fruits and vegetables - contain fiber, especially dried beans and peas and whole grain breads. It is recommended that we consume between 20 to 35 grams of fiber each day.

A great way of cutting fat from our diet is to eliminate meat and increase, vegetables, grains and fruits as your main dish. It is indicated that our daily intake should be less than 30 percent of our total daily calories.

Menopause is the perfect time to begin your future, with your own goal in mind. Approach the second half of your life with vim, vigor, courage, confidence, and conviction.

Remember, fulfillment at midlife is not about age and not about appearance; it is about attitude. There is rich and fertile land on the other side of menopause rite of passage. Welcome the transition and consider it a springboard to a vital, vibrant, and valuable second half of adult life.

Aromatherapy

Many women say that hot flashes are the most troublesome side effect of menopause. Hot flashes happen when blood vessels erratically dilate and constrict. Blood flow increases, body temperature rises, and the heart pumps faster. Sweating usually accompanies hot flashes.

Along with the physical symptoms of menopause, many women experience a fear of growing old, feeling less feminine, or losing their looks. While it is natural to have these concerns, maintaining a bright, optimistic attitude can ease your apprehensions.

A healthy diet, an active lifestyle, and time out for relaxation and stress reduction, can make the transition smoother. Evening Primrose oil and other essential fatty acid supplements provide additional relief for some women. Aromatherapy can diminish many of the discomforts you may experience. Rose, a feminine and nurturing oil, restores confidence, comforts the emotions, and regulates the menstrual cycle. Chamomile oils calms both the body and mind. Clary sage, fennel, geranium, and lavender oils restore hormonal balance. Other essential oils that can help you through menopause are coriander, cypress, jasmine, lavender, orange, patchouli, and ylang ylang.

Below are two aromatherapy blends you can prepare at home.

Menopause Balancing Bath

2 drops chamomile oil
2 drops clary sage oil
2 drops lavender oil
1 drop cypress oil
1 drop fennel oil
1 drop geranium oil

Disperse the essential oils in a bath tub filled with warm water. Soak in the bath for 20 to 30 minutes.

Cool Flash Spray

8 ounces distilled water
4 drops clary sage oil
3 drops chamomile oil
3 drops geranium oil
2 drops cypress oil
1 drop peppermint oil

Combine ingredients in a spray bottle and spritz your face when needed.

Menopause can reduce vaginal secretion and, during this time, one of the best ways to overcome the problem is to continue making love and having orgasms. The amount of vaginal secretion before and during intercourse can vary enormously - largely depending upon our degree of sexual excitement. There are many reasons for the lack of vaginal secretion, such as fright, anxiety, stress and tension. The precise mechanism of the internal vaginal secretion release during the female sexual response is still something of a controversy but clearly relates to hormonal and sexual excitement levels.

The use of nature's essential oils, for whatever purpose, seems to increase the amount of vaginal secretions. Some essential oils seem to increase the supply of vaginal secretion more than others, mainly those that imitate the estrogen hormone. No special treatment is required for this condition - a simple bath or massage oil will do the trick.

Oils for Treating Lack of Vaginal Secretion

Geranium	Sandalwood
Hyacinth	Cinnamon
Rose Bulgar	Lavender
Ylang-Ylang	Nutmeg
Clary Sage	Benzoin
Anise	Savory
Fennel	Cypress
Neroli	Melissa

You can make your own massage oil, using the oils above, by adding 10% of an oil that is good for the skin (borage seed, jojoba, evening primrose, or carrot) to 90% ordinary vegetable oil. Add thirty drops of essential oil to this base mixture of oils, shake gently and apply as you would any body oil, paying attention to the lower abdomen, breasts, and small of the back.

Three Massage Oil Formulas to Overcome Lack of Vaginal Secretion

Geranium	10 drops
Sandalwood	15 drops
Cypress	5 drops
Lavender	10 drops
Neroli	5 drops
Hyacinth	10 drops
Fennel	10 drops
Melissa	4 drops
Clary Sage	15 drops

For baths, the essential oils can be used singularly or in a mixture. Rose Bulgar is a pure indulgent luxury

The Synergistic Blend for Lack of Vaginal Secretion

Rose Bulgar	10 drops
Clary Sage	10 drops
Fennel	2 drops
Hyacinth	2 drops

Mix together into a concentrate, then add 6 drops to each bath.

The Bath Formulas to Overcome Lack of Vaginal Secretion

Rose Bulgar	4 drops
Geranium	2 drops
Cypress	1 drop
Geranium	1 drops
Lavender	2 drops
Hyacinth	2 drops
Melissa	1 drops
Fennel	2 drops
Clary Sage	3 drops

Allow about a week of both daily baths and massage before increased secretion is obtained. Most women find after the third day their vaginas have a nice healthy level of secretion, penetration is easier, and any discomfort, previously experienced by a dry vagina, has gone.

Healing Affirmations

Menopause Problems - Fear of no longer being wanted. Fear of aging. Self-rejection. Not feeling good enough.

Affirmation - I am balanced and peaceful in all changes of cycles, and I bless my body with love.

Abdominal Cramps - Fear. Stopping the process.

Affirmation - I trust the process of life. I am safe.

Aging Problems - Social beliefs. Old thinking. Fear of being one's self. Rejection of the now.

Affirmation - I love and accept myself at every age. Each moment in life is perfect.

Anxiety - Not trusting the flow and the process of life.

Affirmation - I love and approve of myself and I trust the process of life. I am safe.

Apathy - Resistance to feeling. Deadening of the self. Fear.

Affirmation - It is safe to feel. I open myself to life. I am willing to experience life.

Blood Pressure - High – Long standing emotional problem not solved.

Affirmation - I joyously release the past. I am at peace.

Blood Pressure - Low - Lack of love as a child. Defeatism. "What's the use? It won't work anyway?

Affirmation - I now choose to live in the very joyous NOW. My life is a joy.

Breast Problems - A refusal to nourish the self. Putting everyone else first.

Affirmation - I am important. I count. I now care for and nourish myself with love and with joy.

Cataracts - Inability to see ahead with joy. Dark future.

Affirmation - Life is eternal and filled with joy. I look forward to every moment.

Cellulite - Stored anger and self-punishment.

Affirmation - I forgive others. I forgive myself. I am free to love and enjoy life.

Chills - Mental contraction, pulling away and in. Desire to retreat. "Leave me alone."

Affirmation - I am safe and secure at all times. Love surrounds me and protects me. All is well.

Cholesterol - Clogging the channels of joy. Fear of accepting joy.

Affirmation - I choose to love life. My channels of joy are wide open. It is safe to receive.

Circulation - Represents the ability to feel and express the emotions in positive ways.

Affirmation - I am free to circulate love and joy in every part of my world. I love life.

Crying - Tears are the river of life, shed in joy as well as in sadness and fear.

Affirmation - I am peaceful with all of my emotions. I love and approve of myself.

Depression - Anger you feel you do not have a right to have. Hopelessness.

Affirmation - I now go beyond other people's fears and limitations. I create my life.

Fat - Overweight - Over sensitivity. Often represents fear and shows a need for protection. Fear may be a cover for hidden anger and a resistance to forgive.

Affirmation - I am protected by Divine Love. I am always safe and secure. I am willing to grow up and take responsibility for my life. I forgive others and I now create my own life the way I want it. I am safe.

Fat - Arms - Anger at being denied love.

Affirmation - It is safe for me to create all the love I want.

Fat - Belly - Anger at being denied nourishment.

Affirmation - I nourish myself with spiritual food and I am satisfied and free.

Fat - Hips - Lumps of stubborn anger at the parents.

Affirmation - I am willing to forgive the past. It is safe for me to go beyond my parents' limitations.

Fat–Thighs- Packed childhood anger. Often rage at the father.

Affirmation - I see my father as a loveless child and I forgive easily. We are both free.

Fatigue - Resistance, boredom. Lack of love for what one does.

Affirmation - I am enthusiastic about life and filled with energy and enthusiasm.

Female Problems - Denial of the self. Rejecting femininity. Rejection of the feminine principle.

Affirmation - I rejoice in my femaleness. I love being a woman. I love my body.

Frigidity - Fear. Denial of pleasure. A belief that sex is bad. Insensitive partners. Fear of father.

Affirmation - It is safe for me to enjoy my own body. I rejoice in being a woman.

Headaches - Invalidating the self. Self-criticism. Fear

Affirmation - I love and approve of myself. I see myself and what I do with eyes of love. I am safe.

Heart Problems – Long standing emotional problems. Lack of joy. Hardening of the heart. Belief in strain and stress.

Affirmation - Joy. Joy. Joy. I lovingly allow joy to flow through my mind and body and experience.

Indigestion - Gut-level fear, dread, anxiety. Griping and grunting.

Affirmation - I digest and assimilate all new experiences peacefully and joyously.

Insomnia - Fear. Not trusting the process of life. Guilt.

Affirmation - I lovingly release the day and slip into peaceful sleep, knowingly tomorrow will take care of itself.

Left Side of Body - Represents receptivity, taking in, feminine energy, women, the mother.

Affirmation - My feminine energy is beautifully balanced.

Migraine Headaches - Dislike of being driven. Resisting the flow of life. Sexual fears.

Affirmation - I relax into the flow of life and let life provide all that I need easily and comfortably. Life is for me.

Nervousness - Fear, anxiety, struggle, rushing. Not trusting the process of life.

Affirmation - I am on an endless journey through eternity and there is plenty of time. I communicate with my heart. All is well.

Osteoporosis - Feeling there is no support left in life.

Affirmation - I stand up for myself and Life supports me in unexpected, loving ways.

Ovaries - Represent points of creation. Creativity.

Affirmation - I am balanced in my creative flow.

Pain - Guilt. Guilt always seeks punishment.

Affirmation - I lovingly release the past. They are free and I am free. All is well in my heart now.

Right of Body - Giving out. Letting go, masculine, energy, men, the father.

Affirmation - I balance my masculine energy easily and effortlessly.

Sagging Lines - Sagging lines on the face come from sagging thoughts in the mind. Resentment of life.

Affirmation - I express the joy of living and allow myself to enjoy every moment of every day totally. I become young again.

Stomach Problems - Dread. Fear of new. Inability to assimilate the new.

Affirmation - Life agrees with me. I assimilate the new every moment of every day. All is well.

Uterus - Represents the home of creativity.

Affirmation - I am at home in my body.

Yeast Infections - Denying your own needs. Not supporting yourself.

Affirmation - I now choose to support myself in loving, joyous ways

Female Reproductive System

Since the female reproductive system is more complex than its male counterpart, it more often requires the gentle support of herbal remedies. Since ancient times, women have used plant medicines to regulate the women's reproduction organs. Modern scientific analysis confirms the validity of this, since many of the herbal remedies used for these purposes contain steroidal saponins, which closely resemble human hormones.

Menopause marks the end of a woman's child-bearing age. Usually occurring in the early fifties, this is when menstruation ends. Many women experience the change of life with little or no discomfort. Exercising regularly, eating a balanced, whole food diet and leading a happy and full life can help to minimize any discomforts. A drop in estrogen and progesterone can lead some women to experience health problems. These symptoms may include hot flushes, depression, palpitations and a drying up of the natural secretions of the vagina. A mixture of Vitamin E and comfrey ointment can be applied directly to the vagina. Making love regularly contributes to a healthy vagina membrane.

To balance hormones, make a decoction of one part each:

False Unicorn Root
Black Cohosh
Chaste Tree
Blessed Thistle
Wild Yam
Squaw Vine
1/2 part Licorice

Hot flushes can be controlled by drinking a mixed infusion of one teaspoon each of sage and motherwort. Vitamin E (around 400 IU a day) can also help.

For depression, try infusions in equal parts of any one of the following herbs:

Wild Oats
St. John's Wart
Vervain
Borage
Lemon Balm
Motherwort
Rosemary
Skullcap

Palpitations can respond to an infusion of equal parts of:

Valerian
Lemon balm
Hawthorn
Motherwort

Infusions are useful when you want to use the active constituents of a plant that is rich in aromatic oils, if you are using leaves or petals. One part of dried herb is equivalent to three parts fresh.

Infusions are like making a cup of tea. Measure in required amount of herbs and then pour in boiling water, cover and let steep for ten or fifteen minutes.

Decoctions are useful when you are using herbs that are hard and woody. It ensures that the root, bark, or nuts are broken down so that the active ingredients enter the water in solution. Cut up the fresh herbs into small pieces or grind dried ingredients. Measure the required amount into a pan and add water. Bring to boil, cover, and simmer for ten to fifteen minutes. Strain the decoction while still hot.

Chaste Tree
Vitex Agnus Castus
Chasteberry, Monk's Pepper

This plant has a folk use which strongly suggests a hormonal effect. Its Latin and common names seem to suggest that the plant is an anaphrodisiac. In classical times, the plant was used for disorders of the female reproductive system. Research in Germany now indicates that it possesses the ability to increase production of the luteinizing hormone and prolactin. The plant appears to stimulate synthesis of the hormone progesterone. It may also have a regulatory effect on estrogen since herbalists have found it useful for the symptoms of menopause. It has been used to treat fibroids, inflammation of the womb lining, and to reestablish normal ovulation and menstruation after the discontinuation of the contraceptive pill.

Valerian
Valeriana Officinalis

Valerian is an excellent remedy for anxiety, nervous tension, insomnia and headaches. It also has strengthening action on the heart (good for palpitations) along with some indication of lowering blood pressure.

Vervain
Verbena Officinalis

It strengthens the nervous system, dispelling depression and countering nervous exhaustion.

St. John's Wort
Hypericum Perforatum

This herb is used to calm the nervous system and treat depression, particularly during menopause. *This herb can case sensitivity to sunlight.*

Motherwort
Leonurus Cardiccaca
Lion's Tail, Lion's Ear

This herb is used as a sedative particularly valuable in treating the anxiety of menopause. It has the short-term ability to lower blood pressure. Since ancient times, motherwort has been used to treat palpitations and rapid heart beat when associated with anxiety.

Lemon Balm
Melissa Officianlis
Bee Balm, Melissa, Sweet Balm

The great Moslem physician Avicenna recommended this plant because "it makes the heart merry." It is recommended for nervousness, depression, insomnia and nervous headaches. The volatile oils in this plant have a sedative effect even in minute concentrations.

Licorice
Glycyrrhiza Glabra

Licorice is one of the most commonly used herbal remedies because it has the ability to harmonize and blend all the other herbs in a synergy. It can improve the taste of many bitter remedies.

CAUTION: The action of licorice is like that of the hormone of ACTH, causing retention of sodium and potassium and a rise in blood pressure. Avoid licorice if you have high blood pressure or kidney disease or are pregnant. Avoid prolonged use of large doses.

Borage
Borago Officinalis
Bugloss, Burage

Folk use suggests a variety of medicinal properties. It has the ability of counter melancholic states. Pliny repeats an ancient verse, "I, borage always bring courage."

Hawthorn
Crategus Oxyacantha
Mayblossom, Whitehorn

The extraordinary future of this herb is its ability to both, lower high blood pressure and, restore low blood pressure to normal. It is valuable in treating insomnia of nervous origin.

Rosemary
Rosmarinus Officinalis

Rosemary is an excellent remedy for headaches. It also improves the circulation and strengthens fragile blood vessels.

Blessed Thistle
Carduus Benedictus
Holy Thistle, St. Benedict Thistle

Blessed thistle is a diuretic.

Wild Yam
Dioscorea Villosa
Colic Root, Rheumatism Root

It is an antispasmodic action making it useful for treating poor circulation and neuralgia.

Squaw Vine
Mitchella Repens
Partridgeberry, Checkerberry, Deerberry

Not only is the herb a uterine tonic but it also has a calming effect on the nervous system. It improves the digestion.

False Unicorn
Chamaelirium Luteum
Helonias, Blazing Star

False unicorn root contains hormone-like saponins, which account in part of it's considerable reputation as an ovarian and uterine tonic.

Black Cohosh
Cimicifuga Racemosa
Black Snakeroot, Bugbane, Squawroot

Black cohosh, inherited from the Native Americans, is employed for treating headaches and tinnitus. A resinous compound, insoluble in water, lowers blood pressure and dilates the blood vessels. It is an antispasmodic, easing cramping and muscle tension.
CAUTION: This powerful remedy should only to be used by those experienced in herbal medicine. Overdose can result in intense headache, dizziness, visual disturbances, a slow pulse rate, nausea and vomiting. Avoid in pregnancy.

Skullcap

Scutellaria Laterifolia
Helmet Flower, Mad-Dogweed,
Virginian Skullcap

Skullcap is an excellent tonic for the nervous. It is good for treating anxiety, depression, insomnia and nervous headaches.
CAUTION: Large doses may cause dizziness, mental confusion, and erratic pulse rate.

Wild Oats

Avena Sativa

Wild oats, which is harvested in the milky stage, has sexually stimulating effects. It was found up to 200 years ago in the German Pharmacopoeia.

Wild Oats works by freeing up testosterone, the hormone responsible for sex drive, in both males and females. When testosterone is freed from its binding receptors, nature takes it course by stimulating sexual interest in both men and women.

Rejuvenating Female Tonic

This tonic helps maintain and build the body's strength through menopause.

1/2 part borage leaf (maintains adrenal health)
1/2 part lemon balm (lifts spirits)
2 parts fresh raspberry leaf (strengthens female reproductive system)
1 part violet blossom and leaf (tonic to whole system)
1 part burdock root (promotes liver function)
1 part plantain leaf (nourishing and soothing to internal membranes)

Drink as a tea.

Flower Essences

Bottlebrush
Callistemon Linearis

Callistemon means beautiful stamen. These showy bottlebrushes consist of many individual flowers, packed in dense cylindrical spikes, on the tips of the branches.

The bottlebrush essence is for major transitions in life. It helps to give people a belief in their own ability to handle new situations.

There are natural cycles of change in life. Every seven years all our body cells are replaced and, metaphysically, every seven years up to the age of twenty-one another outer body is formed.

Another aspect of this essence is that it helps to brush away the past and allows a person to move on to new situations and experiences. Life is full of ends and beginnings, bringing constant change. To resist change is to block the flow of life.

Positive Outcome:
Serenity and calm
Ability to cope
Ability to move one

Ilawarra Flame Tree
Brachychiton Acerifolius

A mature Flame Tree has thick wrinkled, grey outer bark and lacelike inner bark.

The whole tree blazes as if aflame when in full bloom in early spring.

Because of the properties of this essence, it would not be surprising if the outstretched hand was asking to be accepted.

These people often do things they would rather not, to avoid possible rejection. Such actions are a deep denial of self, and lead to a weakening of the thymus gland, the key to the immune system. Flame Tree essence strengthens and balances the thymus.

These people ignore their potential because they feel overwhelmed by the responsibility of developing it.

Flame Tree remedy will allow them to make a commitment to a certain course of action and they will find the confidence and strength to deal with what they need to do in life, without being overwhelmed by the responsibility of it.

Positive Outcome:
Confidence
Commitment
Strength
Self-reliance
Self-approval

Peach-Flowered Tea-tree
Leptospermum Squarrosum

The shrub bears abundant large, pink blossoms, with five petals, which later turn white. The center of each flower contains nectar. The sweetly scented leaves were used by early sailors to make a tea-like drink. The name Leptospermum refers to the tiny seeds found in the fruit, which is a hard capsule.

The plant is rather ungainly in appearance, with the exception of its attractive flowers.

The Peach-Flowered Tea-Tree is a good remedy for those who lack the will to follow through and for those who have initial enthusiasm that eventually drains away, leaving them without interest.

This remedy is for people who have extreme mood swings and hypochondriacs.

Peach-Flowered Tea-Tree people have vivid imaginations, when it comes to their own health, and are quite convinced they have all sorts of illnesses. Their worries are all related to their bodies. This essence fosters a balanced and responsible attitude towards one's own health, rather than a preoccupation with it.

The change in color of the flower itself indicates its ability to help with mood changes - swings between joy and depression. Peach-Flowered Tea-Tree has a balancing effect on the pancreas. One of the functions of this organ is to control blood sugar levels. It also helps to regulate the kidneys, which control the amount of insulin that the pancreas can provide.

Positive outcome:
Emotional balance
Follow through with projects
Trust in and responsibility for one's own health

She Oak
Casuarina Glaucca

The Casuarinas was one of the first trees to evolve on earth. Its common name, She Oak, came into usage because the early white settlers, who used it's timber for furniture, shingles and house construction, regarded it as the poor man's oak.

The essence is made up using the female flower of the She Oak. Simply adding two drops of this essence to a glass of water will allow an individual to properly absorb and use water. It will regulate the production of reproductive hormones in women, especially where the ovaries are functioning spasmodically, resulting in an irregular menstrual cycle.

In kinesiology, this essence is used to balance the ovaries, and in many cases, it will also balance the testes in men.

Positive outcome:
Hormonal balance
Conception
Fertility

Sexuality

The best way to gain an appreciation of the properties of specific essences, and their relevance to our lives, is to explore a common human theme and to note the essences that are appropriate at various points of that exploration.

An individual's sexuality begins to take shape long before birth. The view is that the emotions present at the time of conception leave a deep impression on the psyche of the child. Indifference, loving passion, drunken rage, terror, or love, whatever is experienced, will be the basic emotion that colors the child's attitude towards the world.

After a break-up of a relationship, Stuart Desert Pea is good if a person is carrying that deep sadness within them. Dagger Hakea can help people deal with the resentment they feel towards the other person. The combination of Bottlebrush and Boronia is excellent for helping them let go of the other person and for healing their broken hearts.

Flannel Flower and Wisteria are essences that can help men and women, respectively, to enjoy sex and closeness. Billy Goat Plum will allow them to experience the beauty of the sexual act and their bodies, especially if they feel unclean after sex.

Our physical reality is created solely by our thoughts and unconscious beliefs.

As individuals age, they pass though major biological transitions such as pregnancy, parenthood, menopause, etc. Bottlebrush will help them cope with these changes, so that they will not feel overwhelmed by them.

As their bodies age, some people lose their self-confidence. These people may want to attract a partner and create a new relationship, yet they hold back because of a lack of confidence in their attractiveness. Five Corners will help to restore their feelings of self-esteem.

Bluebell and Flannel Flower are good remedies for keeping a relationship alive and growing over a long period of time.

Meditation

When you turn inward and find the still center within yourself, you will find the answers to everything you need to know. You will be spiritually, physically and emotionally recharged.

You can create as many rituals as you like around the act of meditating. Burning a candle during meditation, for example, generates a nice energy in the room. Praying directly before meditating is an excellent way to evoke a good feeling in yourself, as well as, a calming protective vibration around you.

It is preferable to meditate approximately the same time each day. Sunrise and sunset are often suitable times for meditating. Choose a time that is most convenient for you.

Twenty minutes is a normal length of time for meditating. Research has shown that twenty minutes of meditation is equivalent to two hours of sleep.

The main purpose of meditation is to still the chatter of the conscious mind, in order to increase your perception of your intuitive nature, and to allow life's dramas and frustrations to fall away or significantly pale.

You could consider your thoughts as clouds. As you become aware of them, do not immediately try to squash them, but rather acknowledge them and then let them simply drift from your awareness.

An important attitude to cultivate towards meditation is to release all expectations. Your higher self, or inner conscious mind, knows exactly what you need, so simply accept whatever happens in meditation as having been chosen by you, in your best interests.

You may find that your sittings are very productive times in which problems are easily solved. Great insight, and understanding, comes through to you.

Bibliography

The 25 Most Important Questions About Menopause by Ruth S. Jacobowitz.

Aromatherapy by Roberta Wilson

Aromantics by Valerie Ann Worwood'

'The New Age Herbalist by Richard Mabey

The Herbal Home Remedy Book by Joyce A. Wardwell

Australian Bush Flower Essences by Ian White

Heal your Body by Louise Hay

Dianne M. Kapral, N.D., R.H.A., received her doctorate from The Clayton College of Natural Health. She received her registration for Hypno-Anesthesiology from the National Board of Hypno-Anesthesiology (NBHA). She founded Peak Performance Unlimited to help people achieve their own peak performance through mind/body awareness. Through skilled hypnotherapy, Dr. Kapral effectively replaces crystallized negative habits, fears and tension with positive suggestions and a sense of relaxation in her clients. The results are a well-aligned individual who is readily able to rely on the body's natural painkillers and stress relievers.

Working with doctors and dentists, Dr. Kapral helps their patients alleviate anxiety, fear and pain. Her practice also includes work in areas of stress, weight and pain management, smoking cessation, exercise and sales motivation, goal obtainment, sports enhancement, overcoming phobias and procrastination and increasing concentration, study habits and memory recall.

Using her knowledge, she has assisted women with a pain-free, stress-free childbirth, using herbs, relaxation techniques and Aromatherapy.

Dr. Kapral conducts seminars for private and professional groups.

Her motto is: *What the mind perceives, the body achieves.*

You may reach Dr. Kapral through her email address: dmkapral@msn.com. Or her web site: http://mysite.verizon.net/res7jrno/diannekapralnd

Notes

Notes

Notes

www.ingramcontent.com/pod-product-compliance
Lightning Source LLC
Chambersburg PA
CBHW050345290526
45785CB00006B/2642